Delusion of Theft in Dementia

Landa George

ISBN-10: 1541339371
ISBN-13: 978-1541339378

DEDICATION

"We can complain because rose bushes have thorns, or rejoice because thorn bushes have roses" Abraham Lincoln

This book is dedicated to my mother Essie whose disability and vulnerabilities has helped me to develop resilience, empathy, patience and my strong family values. I used to pray so hard that mum's hearing would come back, however now I understand that the challenges and obstacles we face in life, are our opportunities to develop emotional muscle and strength of character. That has been her gift to me. Thanks mum.

CONTENTS

Landa George

ACKNOWLEDGMENTS

I would like to acknowledge my husband Colin and my children Cory, Jayden and Maleika for giving me quiet time during the research, planning, writing, editing and formatting for this book. Thanks for being patient when the "Mum's working!" sign was up and I was up in my office (my bedroom) writing this book instead of spending quality time with you all, my beloved family.

Essie story

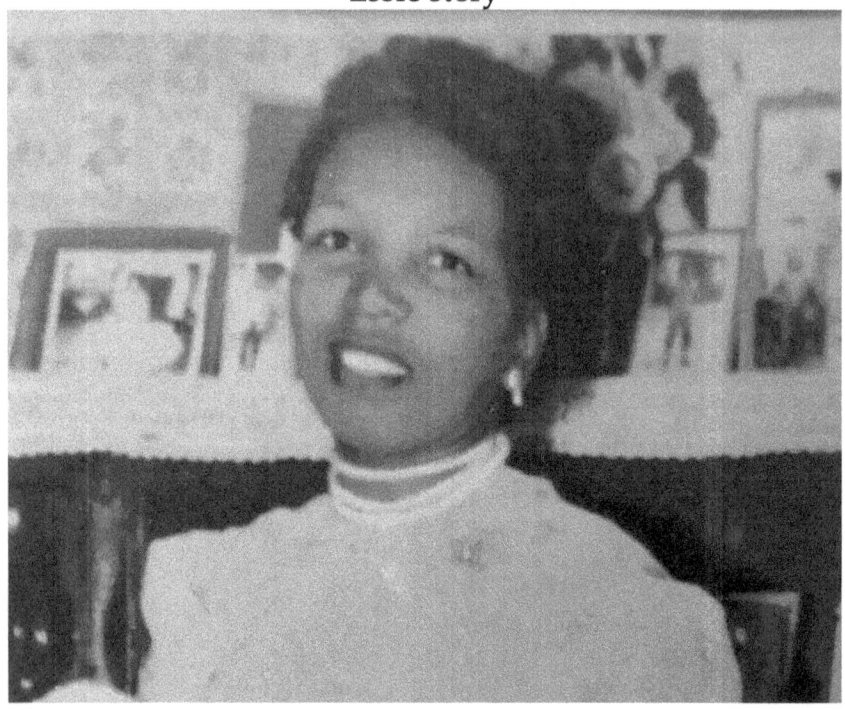

1 WHY I WROTE THIS BOOK

"I bought a big bottle of olive oil and Mimi took it. No matter what I buy, sugar, coffee, she takes it! I'm not telling no lies"
Essie

This book was primarily inspired by a desire to support my mum to have peace of mind and feel safe. During the last ten years, I have seen my mother change from a loving, friendly, independent older person to someone who is paranoid, frightened, isolated and vulnerable. I believed at one time that only my mum was experiencing these distressing paranoid thoughts called delusions of theft. Now I know there are others who are similarly misunderstood and stigmatized.

Since my mum's first delusions started to surface in the late 1990's, I have seen family members create distance between them and my mum because they are unable to cope with her challenging beliefs and behaviours. This has caused fragmentation in our family that will never be healed. My mum has grandchildren and great grandchildren she will never be close to and it is mostly as a result of her delusions. In writing this book, my goal is to share what works and what doesn't work, for carers and families of those with delusions. I would like to save carers from experiencing the years of trial and error my family have been through and reduce the impact of delusions of theft on their loved ones. By putting in place the strategies outlined in this book, the quality of care for your loved one will increase and the stress and frustration experienced by carers will decrease.

The idea for this book developed throughout the end of 2015 during my own search for solutions when my mother's delusions were at their most intense, and my aim is to share my knowledge and experience to help others. If I can do that, then I will be very happy.

I always believe it is best to start at the beginning, so a little bit about my mum. She was born Esther but will be referred to by her nickname Essie from this point on in this book.

Essie was born on a small island in the Caribbean called Montserrat, and when I say a small island, I mean a really small island! You can drive around it in one hour and in the days when Essie grew up there everyone knew everyone else and was probably related to everyone else somewhere along the line, as there was only about 12,000 inhabitants.

However in 1997, Montserrat was devastated by a volcanic eruption that changed the landscape, the people and the lifestyle of those living there forever. Now it is even quicker to circumference the island as it has been divided into three areas to protect people in the event of further volcanic eruption. The area which has the highest risk just below the volcano is a "no go zone". There is an area where people can visit only in the day, the "daytime zone" and there is the "safe zone" where all inhabitants live.

There are now only about 5,000 people on Montserrat, as many people who had lived there all their lives were forced to flee. They were evacuated and taken in as refugees by neighbouring islands, the USA, Canada and the UK.

After arriving in the UK in 1958, it was always Essie's dream to retire back to Montserrat - her green and luscious island with lots of sun, fresh vegetation, warm and friendly people. She had just finished building her retirement home in 1997 high up on the mountain, when the eruption began. She tells me her home was beautiful. She describes how the veranda was wrapped around three sides of the house so she could get a cool breeze while overlooking the ocean, lush greenery and the pink and purple bougainvillea flowers so plentiful on the island. However, nature had other ideas and this dream has now been abandoned.

Essie was the eldest and bossiest child born into a farming family in the 1930's. She lived with her father, mother and five younger siblings- four brothers and one sister. Her parents grew their own food and sold surplus products in the town's market for their income. Essie and her family experienced poverty growing up but no-one ever was hungry with fresh, organic produce galore on the trees and in the land. Life was mostly good.

Everything changed for Essie drastically however when she was 12 years old when she contracted a disease called Typhoid. She was very unwell in the hospital with a high fever for several days and her family thought that she may die. The doctors tried everything they could to save her and so administered a drug called Quinine that they thought would break her fever. It worked, Essie's fever came down. However, the side effects of the drug resulted in damage to the nerves in her inner ears, resulting in permanent and substantial hearing loss.

From that moment, Essie would never hear her siblings call her name or her baby sister's laughter ever again. I mourn for that little 12 year old girl whose education and childhood ended right there. Due to the size of Montserrat, there was a lack of specialised resources and in a time when the world was at war it probably was not a priority. Considering this time in Essie's life makes me look at my children and think how it would affect them to be suddenly cut off from the world, school, conversations, jokes, music, TV and laughter, permanently.

In her twenties, Essie got an opportunity to come to the UK to explore medical interventions that could restore some of her hearing. She left her two year old daughter, Rosanna, in the care of her sister and mother and embarked on a six week voyage on a huge ship across the Atlantic Ocean. Essie tells me that she endured motion and seasickness every single day of that long voyage but that everyone abroad helped and supported each other. Through that experience, she made friends for life.

Once in England and after medical investigations, Essie was offered an operation that doctor thought would help restore some of her hearing. However, it would involve invasive surgery to her skull to operate on her auditory nerves. However, Essie's father had died as a result of complications following surgery on his prostrate and this scared Essie. After considering her options, Essie decided that she was not willing to take a chance of something going wrong and declined the operation. Essie decided to make the best of her life as it was and she did.

Essie lived, worked and made a life for herself in the UK. She got married, had three more children, two boys and one girl and later divorced. She sent for Rosanna (Rosie) when she was 13, but due to the period of separation that had lapsed between Essie's voyage when Rosanna was 2 year old, they never rekindled the close mother daughter bond that could have been. Her sons Lloyd and Trevor were the middle children and then there was me, youngest daughter. Due to Essie's physical disability and low literacy skills, I have always been her main carer and advocate. So in fitting with my role, I am writing the story of her Dementia as I know it.

When this story intensified for us, Essie was 84 years old and had been diagnosed with Vascular Dementia for five years. She lived on her own in a one bedroom bungalow and was fairly independent. She loved to visit her local market, social club, friends, family, and church on a weekly basis. She was independent with her shopping, cleaning and personal care.

However, in 2014 she began to need more support as she became frailer following a bout of the flu and so we asked her neighbour Mimi to provide paid cleaning for a few hours per week as she lives opposite. Mimi had provided unpaid care and support to Essie over a period of 15 years, first as a volunteer and then gradually Essie had grown to become a member of her extended family.

Mimi and her family's culturally background is African. They have strong family values and so virtually adopted Essie. Over a period of 18 years Essie became "CoCo Essie" or "CoCo Esther" which is a term of endearment, as she was like a grandmother figure to Mimi's four small children. For a long time the arrangement was mutually beneficial.

At the time, we were aware that Essie had delusional thinking about her eldest daughter Rosanna (Rosie). It was intensive, relentless and had been focussed on Rosanna for about 10 years. I was so accustomed to that status quo I didn't expect her delusional thoughts would be transferred to anyone else. I thought there was minimal risk to Mimi as she was so loved and such a central part of Essie's support system, but I was wrong.

Our paid arrangement with Mimi worked brilliantly for a few months. Mimi knew Essie, was able to communicate with her and they got on really well. Our family trusted Mimi and we could see both parties were benefiting from the arrangement. However, in early 2015 something started to change. Essie started voicing concerns that Mimi was stealing household items- clothing, curtains, pots and utensils and food items. Initially, most our family ignored these allegations because we knew they were ridiculous. However, as the allegations become more detailed some in our family stated to question whether these thefts were taking place.

We considered every logical scenario- maybe someone did have a key, maybe Essie was losing her belongings in the house, or maybe Mimi really was taking things? We decided that no, Mimi was not taking things. We could see Essie was becoming increasingly agitated and we started to suspect that she just wasn't very well. We had grown to know Mimi well over the years and knew the allegations were false. We all tried to convince Essie that Mimi had done nothing wrong.

However, our efforts were in vain. Essie had an unshakeable belief that Mimi was stealing from her and grew frustrated and angry that her children were not taking action.

Each visit became a battle ground. Essie became upset, distressed and tearful as she was not being taken seriously. She honestly believed Mimi was coming in and taking her household items and this made Essie her feel vulnerable and paranoid. The situation affected Essie's sleep and she felt anxious all the time. Each time we visited we argued on Mimi's behalf and Essie argued against, we were locked into a cycle of allegations, defence, conflict and heated arguments.

Every visit become stressful and unpleasant and as a result certain family members avoided visits to Essie. The impact was that Essie become more isolated and feel even more vulnerable.

After many requests, we changed Essie's locks and this made her feel secure for a week or so. However, within weeks, she wanted her locks changed again. Her accusations continued and grew more intense with each passing week.

With my background in mental health nursing, I was worried and concerned that as Essie's behaviour was becoming more and more chaotic. She was putting herself at risk and self-isolating which in turn had a negative effect on her mood.

Then on a Sunday in late 2015, I arrived at Essie's home to take her to church and she was in a fury. She was angry, ranting and was more agitated than I had ever seen her before. Her eyes wild, she accused Mimi of entering her home and taking sugar, again. She refused to go to church because she believed Mimi would come in and steal while she was out. I couldn't calm her down, I couldn't distract her. I had never seen her like that before and I was worried about her physical and mental health. I eventually left her and went to church about five minutes' drive away.

However, during service I couldn't get Essie off my mind. I Had never seen her so angry and distressed. So I left the church service early and telephoned the out of hours mental health team for advice. Hanging on the telephone line that Sunday, I was worried and troubled about what the future held for Essie. Was this the beginning of the end? Was this a crossroads towards Essie needing more assistance and possibility towards residential care? I was told there was no emergency mental health assessment team for over 65 year olds so Essie would have to be referred to the older adults mental health team via her doctor.

On the following day, I called and explained the developing situation to Essie's doctor who made a referral to the mental health team for older adults. Within a few weeks, a psychiatrist visited and after a thorough assessment confirmed Essie was experiencing delusions of theft and reviewed her medication.

Essie had been on a small dosage of Quetiapine since her diagnosis of Vascular Dementia five years previously and so it was recommended to slightly increase her Quetiapine. Reluctantly, I agreed and this change was updated in her medication within the next week.

Despite a slight increase in Essie's Quetiapine, the change caused chaos. Perhaps it was the fact that Essie had been on the same level of medication for so many years but soon after the being on the higher dosage, Essie complained of hearing "music". In my mind I expected this would be a pleasant experience, but Essie found the noise or "music" distressing after no hearing for 62 years. The "music" disturbed her sleep, she became fretful, irritable, upset and tearful. The change in medication was not working and had in fact made the situation worse.

Following an emergency assessment of Essie's medication, the psychiatrist recommended a change from Quetiapine to Risperidone. This new suggestion concerned me because of the possibility of increased side effects. Would it make the situation worse? However, despite my concerns the situation felt desperate. After speaking to my siblings I reluctantly agreed to a change to Risperidone. The next few months of experimentation were a nightmare for Essie, Mimi and our family. Essie was in tears every time we visited and complained she couldn't sleep because of all the worry. There were now regular verbal altercations between Essie and Mimi initiated by Essie. In the space of a few weeks Essie gained entry and searched Mimi's home in the early hours of the morning. Police had been called to an argument involving Essie and Mimi in the street. The surrounding neighbours were complaining that Essie was shouting at home when alone. The neighbours avoided Essie due to her aggressive demeanour and paranoid ramblings. Family members now either avoided visiting or cut their visits short as they were worn down by Essie's accusations and threats to go the police about Mimi. We grew more and more impatient with the accusations and erratic behaviours and there were suggestions from some family members that Essie could no longer continue to live independently due to her delusional thinking.

In the early hours of the morning, one night while I was struggling to sleep and worrying about Essie and how we were going to continue support her, I googled "accusations of theft" on my phone. In a few short minutes, my outlook on Essie's illness and our situation completely changed forever. In my search online, I came across an American forum where carers were talking about their elderly relatives delusions. I was both astounded and relieved at the same time! The behaviours, the difficulties, the allegations, the responses of their loved ones were so similar to Essie, that I felt I was reading about her. I felt at last that we were not alone and other people understood what we were going through. Other carers were experiencing what my family were experiencing. They had the same issues we had and possibly had some answers on how we could manage this situation better. At last I felt there was hope. I now felt motivated to find strategies that would calm Essie, give her peace of mind and assist her to remain independent for as long as possible. I decided that whatever I found, I would share with as many carers and families who have loved ones experiencing delusions of theft as I could. For all those struggling with this issue, this book is for you.

2 WHAT ARE DELUSIONS?

"She is stealing my curtains and that's why I took them out to count them. There are 12 of them. If she wants curtains she should buy them" Essie

Delusions are strongly held false beliefs or thoughts that have no basis in reality. These delusions remain in place despite attempts to convince the person otherwise from family, friends or professionals and despite all evidence to the contrary.

Paranoid delusions are irrational thoughts that bad things are happening and that certain people are responsible. People experiencing paranoid delusions can have a variety of beliefs that are persecutory in nature, for example that someone is trying to poison them or watching them. Paranoid beliefs are extremely distressing to the person, as they absolutely believe them to be true. They are especially upset if their loved ones, and most trusted friends and family don't believe them. These delusions are unshakable despite any evidence being presented that their beliefs are unlikely, unreasonable or just plain impossible! Delusions that someone is stealing, taking belongings or replacing personal items with substitutes, is one of those paranoid delusions.

Sometimes it is difficult for carers to understand the extent to an unshakeable belief. They believe that if they can provide indisputable evidence, that the person with Dementia will suddenly see the error of their thinking. We have now had nearly 20 years of trying this strategy and it has been my experience that attempting to convince or dispute the belief does not work.

It was more than a decade ago now, that Essie had visited the bank to deposit some savings. When she arrived back home she looked at her deposit book and realised something was wrong and a mistake had been made. I arrived home one afternoon to encounter a very upset Essie outside my front door waiting for me.

She explained that she had gone to the bank that afternoon to deposit some cash and that it was only when she had returned home and checked her deposit book that she realised that no funds had been added to her account. Essie believed that the cashier had pretended to deposit the cash in her account but then kept the cash. I examined the savings book but there was no deposit for that day. I had no proof of what had happened either way but Essie was convinced of her version of the story.

Although I felt it was unlikely, I had no proof to the contrary and so I supported her to make a formal complaint to the police. The police investigation was thorough.

They scrutinized the camera recordings and then they came back to me. They advised that Essie had been in the bank that day as she had said. Essie had also been in the queue but she had left the bank before being serviced by the cashier. Essie had not deposited any funds onto her account that day. We never found out where the money disappeared to but most importantly, despite what the police and the video evidence said, Essie was firm in her belief that the cashier was a thief. After many requests, I supported Essie to close her account and move her savings to another bank. She will always claim the cashier stole her money, whatever the cashier, police or video evidence ever says.

"I remember long ago, we called the police on Essie's behalf. When the police came they said "we can't see anywhere the thief has entered, unless it was a ghost" This was when she was saying things were getting lost, so at that time the police came to search, they looked and could not see anything to confirm that a thief had entered the house. The police said it must be because she is old or it must be ghosts because no one else has entered the house" Mimi

3 PRESENTATION OF DELUSIONS OF THEFT

"That bitch came and took it!" Essie

Delusions that people are stealing is the most common delusion experienced by people with Dementia and is commonly known as delusion of theft. Although delusions of theft can be experienced by those with other psychotic illness such as schizophrenia, in this book I will be focussing on people who have an underlying diagnosis of Dementia or Alzheimer's disease.

For most people who experience delusion of theft as a result of Dementia, it comes with a loss of independence due to reduced function which requires support from others on a regular basis. Perhaps as a result, accusations of theft are normally aimed at relatives, loved ones, neighbours and primary carers either formal or informal. Relatives and carers who provide intensive physical or emotional support can find themselves on the wrong end of accusations that they are stealing items from the cared for person. This can be stressful, confusing and hurtful for the accused and Mimi impact on their ability to provide quality of care. In families, accusations can prove to be divisive, especially when some family members believe false accusations. Believing the deluded person is understandable, because people with delusions are so convicted and convincing that people who know them well, have no reason to doubt their claims. The end result Mimi be split allegiances and families torn apart into those believing a theft has occurred and those refuting any incidence at all.

"At one stage yes, I believed her. The reason I believed her was, it was too many coincidences. Too many things going missing over a period of time. I thought maybe someone was preying on the old woman and they had a key. maybe they were coming in and maybe instead of ransacking the place, just taking the odd thing so they could come back a month later and take something else" Lloyd

Many items that are believed to be stolen are of low value and are normal household items. These may include clothing, pots, cutlery, documents, sugar, washing powder, cheese, shampoo, cream, personal items such as teeth, glasses and wigs. However, valuable items are also claimed to be stolen such as jewellery and cash. In reality, most items have been lost or hidden somewhere in the home for safe keeping by the person who is suffering from impaired memory or feelings of insecurity. The person experiencing Dementia may want to put items away for safe keeping however as a result of memory difficulties they may promptly forget where they have hidden them.

Many carers report that people experiencing delusion of theft can have most usual hiding places. Essie hides a collection of scissors and other sharp objects under the sofa. I have no idea why, but at least I know where to go if I need a screwdriver.

"She accused me and said I took rings and watches and we found the rings in the cabinet in the small drinking glasses, the rings were in there" Rosie

With the progression of Dementia, recognition skills become impaired and those with Dementia can fail to recognise items that may have been in their possession for years. They may then express concerns that someone has taken and replaced their belongings with alternative items. Essie currently has many of her pots and pans on her kitchen floor. She says the pots and pans are not hers and that Mimi took hers and replaced them. She refuses to use theses pots and cannot give a logical explanation why Mimi would exchange her pots and pans. She also believes that Mimi has entered into her home and left a selection of tea-shirts and clothes that are not hers. Essie is really mad about this! Recently, Essie brought out a whole pile of clothes and went into a rant that was very difficult to stop. As evidence of the replacement of her clothes Essie explained how each item was either much too big or too small for her and then proceeded to throw them on the floor with distain.

One of the coping strategies a person with Dementia may have is to buy many of the same items as a response to the loss that is experienced when items go missing or are assumed to be stolen. This may make the person with Dementia feel initially more secure emotionally but on a practical level an increase of items in the home due to stockpiling can result in an increased difficultly locating other items; this may then trigger more accusations that someone has been taking things. Essie has a long history of stockpiling or hoarding behaviour. Some experts believe hoarding is more likely to happen in older adults who have had experience of poverty or lack in their life time and due to Essie's early years growing up in a farming family in the war years this may be true for her.

As a social worker working with psychotic service users, in 2015 I worked with an older person who was from a former eastern bloc country who hoarded books. She explained to me one day that when she was young she loved reading and was passionate about books. However, some books were very expensive at that time and had to be smuggled into her country. Therefore, when she arrived in the UK she was able to indulge herself and buy as many books as she wanted and so she did, hundreds of them. However, because of the perceived value held from her childhood, she was never able to throw or give any books away. This led her to being almost buried in hundreds and hundreds of books in her small flat.

Essie does not hoard books, but she has an obsession about sports tea-shirts. She has over one hundred of them, in every colour, stripped and multi-coloured. She has about seven suitcases in her bedroom to accommodate these and various clothes items she purchased in preparation for her emigration back to Montserrat. She had until recently, so many suitcases that there was no space to sleep on her bed.

In addition to the cognitive causes of accusations, the combination of memory loss and environmental factors may make it more difficult to locate items. It is thought that a person with Dementia misplaces an item in their home and then creates a 'story' to make sense of the lost item. This 'story' usually denies any possibility of memory issues and puts the blame firmly on someone close to them who they believe has the opportunity to take the item.

The person experiencing delusions of theft can be angry, upset, tearful, agitated and scared about the items they believe have been taken. They maybe be frustrated and exasperated when they are not believed or taken seriously. They are likely to want action either to expose, embarrass or confront the "thief" and in many cases will demand that the police are called so that charges can be brought. This can be a difficult and complex situation if the main carer is the person accused, as it can lead to increased isolation for the person suffering from delusion of theft when they refuse to allow their carer into their home or refuse to talk to them. The person experiencing delusions can become more and more threatening and challenging at every encounter.

Aggressive and violent behaviour is always a possibility with delusion of theft due to the high level of feelings evoked when the sufferer truly believes that they have been victimised by someone they trust. They feel a sense of injustice and betrayal at what has occurred and this gives raise to powerful feelings.

"When she is upset, she moves her hands, she is really loud and it is scary. It is scary the way she fights. Up to now she is doing it. If I have to go to her house, I listen from the kitchen window and she is fighting with herself" Litsa

4 EFFECT ON CARERS

"I don't want her back here! She is a thief! I'm going to report her to the police!" Essie

Due to the emotional impact, those who care for a relative or loved one with delusions of theft are at increased risk of developing anxiety, depression and feelings of guilt and loss. Carers are vulnerable to social pressure and stigma about their loved one's behaviour which can affect their physical health and cause psychological distress. This ongoing and relentless stress on the carer, ultimately impacts the care they are providing to the person with Dementia.

Most carers who provide care for those suffering from delusions of theft are informal carers and have a connection with the cared for person, either being a spouse, relative, friend or neighbour. Many provide unpaid care and make sacrifices in order to support their loves ones. Caring can be physically, mentally and emotionally draining, as well as impacting on work and finances. To add to that the additional pressure of accusations of theft can be overwhelming for a carer, especially if they find themselves the person "accused". Many carers are likely to take things personally and be offended that their loved one could believe that the incidence ever occurred. Other carers will just ignore accusations, expecting delusions to be short term and wait for all to return to normal. However, if the situation fails to rectify itself in a short space of time, carers may feel a range of emotions including frustration or even anger, believing that the person with Dementia is just being difficult or vindictive. Any historic relational issues will make the situation more hurtful and painful for the carer which can become a barrier to carers providing sensitive and appropriate care.

"After that I realised something was wrong with her. She accused me of lots of different things, but by that time I had stopped talking to her. I decided I would not go back to her house. When someone comes and accuses you, you keep your distance" Rosie

The long-term result may be that many carers find themselves unable to take the barrage of accusations, insults and emotional trauma involved in being around their loved ones. They may eventually withdraw emotionally and sometimes withdraw their support physically by relocating or ending their caring role. The burden of caring for someone with delusion of theft and the impact of any reduction in support from carers may be a factor in earlier admittance to residential care for an older person due to emotional burnout of the main carer. If the person with Dementia remains in the community however, delusions of this kind can put people with Dementia at an increased risk of abuse. A study of carers in 1993 suggested that carers experiencing abuse from those suffering from Dementia were at a higher risk of being abusive back. This study suggested that there was a relationship between the high psychological and physical demands placed on carers and elder abuse.

Carers that continue to care during episodes of delusions of theft have reported feeling a high level of stress, experiencing low mood and insomnia and even feeling suicidal. Carers can feel isolated and scapegoated especially if accusations are believed by family and community. Just when a supportive network is most needed, family and support networks can be negatively impacted with people taking sides of who they believe is telling the truth. In my family, the first person to be targeted on a consistent basis was my older sister, Rosie. Essie accused Rosie of stealing plates, clothes and hats for years. Watching close hand, I know these accusations have been deeply hurtful for Rosie and have had a negative impact on her relationship with her mother despite her understanding of Dementia.

"My daughter Kandaze was about 9 or 10 years old and I remember her running up and down the corridor crying. I remember Kandaze crying and I was thinking, look at what the child is seeing. From that day, she couldn't really get close to her grandmother. It affected her relationship with her grandmother because her grandmother was making all that noise. She was seeing her mum so upset and all over plates" Rosie

5 CAUSES AND RISK FACTORS

"I'm not stupid" She keeps stealing, stealing my clothes. All my clothes. She goes with them and sells them" Essie

Behavioural and psychological symptoms or BPSD are a group of symptoms experienced by people with Dementia. These symptoms can be expressed as agitation, aggression, depression, shouting, hallucinations or delusions. One of the most common symptoms of BPSD are paranoid delusions, with delusions of theft being the most common paranoid delusion experienced by those affected by Dementia. In the UK today we have approximately 850,000 people diagnosed with Dementia, so the potential number of people and carers affected by delusion of theft is large and growing.

According to the Faculty of the psychiatry of Old Age, BPSD such as delusions of theft are a "complex interaction of the illness, the environment, physical health, medication and interaction with others". There is no single clear cause or explanation for delusion of theft, but there are three main possibilities. The first one is that delusions are caused by brain damage or imbalance caused by Dementia which causes cognitive decline and result in memory loss, disorientation or confusion. The second explanation is that delusions may be caused by a separate disorder unrelated to Dementia or environmental factors. Lastly, an explanation may be that delusions are a response to inadequacies in the environment and social factors which react with the physical and cognitive restrictions posed by their Dementia. This last explanation fits in with my experiences. I believe delusions of theft are an interaction between Dementia and environmental and social factors. So in this section, I will explore some environmental and social factors and how these may affect the development of delusions of theft.

As we age, the environment which may have met our needs when we were younger may no longer be appropriate for us because of the deterioration in our physical bodies and our cognitive processes. In addition to this, most people also experience reduced social contact as they become less active, retire from work, children move away and spouses die. It is likely that this combination of increased needs, inadequate environments, reduced social stimulation along with a diagnosis of Dementia, may have a negative impact on our ability to function, reduce our quality of life and be a trigger for delusion of theft.

Delusion of theft may be triggered initially after a person cannot locate personal items or valuables. Although decline in cognitive function is a major factor, the loss of an item may be linked to environmental influences like poor lighting in conjunction with physical issues like failing eyesight. Research suggests that by the time we are 65 years old we need 3 times more light than when we are in our 20's, and by the time we are 85 years old we need about 5 times as much light. Therefore, as we age and our eyesight deteriorates, our environment should be adapted to provide improved quality lighting. However, most people are unaware of this deterioration and make no adaptation in the environment of older people and when planning care. A study in 2011 on delusions in Dementia (Cohen-Mansfield) found that participants with delusions were more likely to have poorer vision and hearing. It found that sensory difficulties were a risk factor in delusion of theft developing. It does seem logical that the increased vulnerability of aging, fragility along with a decline in memory, hearing and sight may contribute to the development of this delusion. This is a sound assumption in Essie's case. She has become more paranoid and displayed more intense delusions, as she became more physically frail and her eyesight has deteriorated with age.

In the last few months, we have found out that Essie has substantial cataracts in both eyes which may have developed over a number of years. These deteriorations in her physical health alongside her substantial sensory loss put her at a higher risk of developing a delusion.

Another environmental factor which may feed into the development of a delusion of theft is the issue of hoarding. Hoarding is the compulsion to acquire items or the inability to throw out items which may be of insignificant value to others. Hoarding occurs for many reasons, but for older people with Dementia, it seems to be associated with a fear of loss. Hoarding is a strategy for a person with Dementia to feel more secure and to ensure against scarcity. Hiding items in the home environment or hoarding items helps them to feel safe and may be a sort of insurance policy against lack for those who experienced poverty in their life time. However, hoarding can cause significant environmental concerns that can lead to health and safety issues like increase risk of falls. fire or pest control issues. In addition, the habit of hoarding in conjunction with impaired memory and declining eyesight may leave older people unable to locate items in a home that is disorganised and cluttered. The frustration and stress of trying to locate items in less than favourable environmental circumstances could then be a trigger for the forming of a delusion that someone close has stolen the item they are looking for. This scenario may not be the case for your loved one, but it may be helpful to consider what environmental factors might increase risk factors and make their home situation more difficult.

Whilst researching for this book, the positive effects of social contact was also identified as important in the issue of delusion of theft. Researchers exploring risk factors in delusion of theft by Murayama in 2009 found that people living alone showed significantly more frequent delusion of theft than people living with their families. It is suggested that the lower risk enjoyed by those with Dementia living within a family unit may be due to family support searching for items, however it could also be as a result of more social contact. We will never know what the protective factor was in that study but I do know that since we have put into place daily visiting schedule for Essie we have found that she has become calmer and although her delusions are still present they seem to be less distressing for her.

6 TREATMENT OPTIONS

"They're not mine! They're not mine! I'm not stupid!" Essie

Dementia is a degenerative disease which affects cognitive functions such as memory, thinking, behaviour and the ability to perform everyday activities. Despite being associated with older people and the aging process, it is not a normal part of aging.

As the world's population ages, there is a commitment to find a find a cure or drug therapy to help with the side effects of Dementia. In the world today, there are over 47.5 million people living with Dementia. It is estimated that by 2030 that number would have increased to 75.6 million and this figure will be an extraordinary 135.5 million by 2050. This number represents disability and dependency for those affected but also a huge impact for carers and society as a whole. Seeing this ticking time bomb approaching, scientists worldwide are searching for a cure, however, there is no current cure for Dementia or pharmaceuticals that will halt its progression.

A delusion of theft is a Behavioural and Psychological Symptoms of Dementia (BPSD) and studies consistently show that BPSD's are one of the most significant symptoms experienced by people with Dementia. BPSD presents differently for each individual and symptoms can reduce and disappear over a period of time or become more severe and progressive. It is when symptoms become severe or distressing for sufferers and carers that expertise may be sought from a doctor.

There are very few pharmacological treatments for delusions of theft except antipsychotics (drugs developed to treat schizophrenia). The antipsychotics currently used are Risperidone, Olanzapine and Quetiapine. Only Risperidone is licensed for BPSD and it is used along with Olanzapine and Quetiapine to reduce BPSD symptoms. There are disagreements over the effectiveness and safety of these medicines and concerns that they can cause cognitive decline and increase risks of strokes. However, a small study in 2002 (published in the International Journal of Geriatric Psychiatry) selected only adults experiencing delusion of theft. Results claimed to have a positive outcome for reducing and eliminating symptoms using Risperidone. As a result, this study claimed that carer stress was significantly reduced. Conversely, there have also been other studies disputing the effectiveness of antipsychotics and highlighting health concerns over serious side effects including increased risk of strokes, blood clots and falls. As a result of health concerns and conflicts in opinions, psychiatrists are more reluctant to prescribe anti-psychotic medications unless BPSD is severe.

Conflicts in opinions of experts can make decision making very difficult for carers and I empathize with any carers currently facing decisions about treatment options. I cannot advise on the best course of action, I can only share our journey in 2015. It was a very difficult decision to change Essie's medication from Quetiapine which she had been taking for 5 years without any issues to Risperidone. We did not want to expose her to higher risks posed by Risperidone, however on a day to day basis we could see the distress she was experiencing and that she had virtually no quality of life.

Eventually, we made the decision that we felt was the best for Essie. You will have to weigh up the risks versus the benefits in your loved one's case and make the decision you believe is in their best interest. The only suggestion I would make would be to attempt implementing the life style changes I have outlined in section three first, to see if they reduce the occurrences of delusions for the person you care for.

"I think she has an imaginary friend and it's her way of dealing with her situation and having someone to talk to even though there is no one there. It is her way of getting her frustrations out Maybe"
Lloyd

7 ARE DELUSIONS OF THEFT COMMON?

"She should take her money and buy what she wants. Plenty things she has taken from me. I'm fed up with her!" Essie

There is a growing awareness in the media about issues relating to Dementia and care, however despite the growing awareness and the large percentage of people experiencing delusion of theft there is limited public awareness of the emotional turmoil that carers experience when they are caring for someone with a fixed delusion of this kind.

Until late in 2015, I thought our family's situation and Essie's fixation was unusual. I was not aware of anyone with parents who had paranoid thoughts about people coming in and stealing from them. I had never heard about delusions of theft in the media and this made me feel like we were isolated and experiencing this challenges alone.

I qualified as a mental health nurse in 2013 and worked with older adults with Dementia and challenging behaviour for three months whilst on placement and it was never highlighted as a common delusion. It was only when I started working with people with schizophrenia that these particular paranoid thoughts introduced to me and I was able to draw striking similarities between the two presentations of delusions of theft.

In the next decade, I believe that awareness of the issues surrounding delusions of theft will increase, because as we live longer, the number of older adults experiencing Dementia will increase.

Last year in 2016 in the UK 850,000 people were suffering from Dementia and it is believed that the number affected by Dementia in the UK will go up to 1 million by 2020. It is believed that between 10-70% of people with Dementia experience delusions, with delusion of theft being the most common type of delusion. Therefore, the number of adults affected by delusion of theft will significantly increase in the next 5 years.

"I had heard of other people with this illness. My friend Yvonne, her mum was the same. Her mum used to say that she stole things. Yvonne didn't live there but when she went there, her mum was always missing something. She didn't accuse the others; she would always say Yvonne had taken it. Yvonne was the oldest and she lived away from her mum. They didn't have a particularly good relationship" Rosie

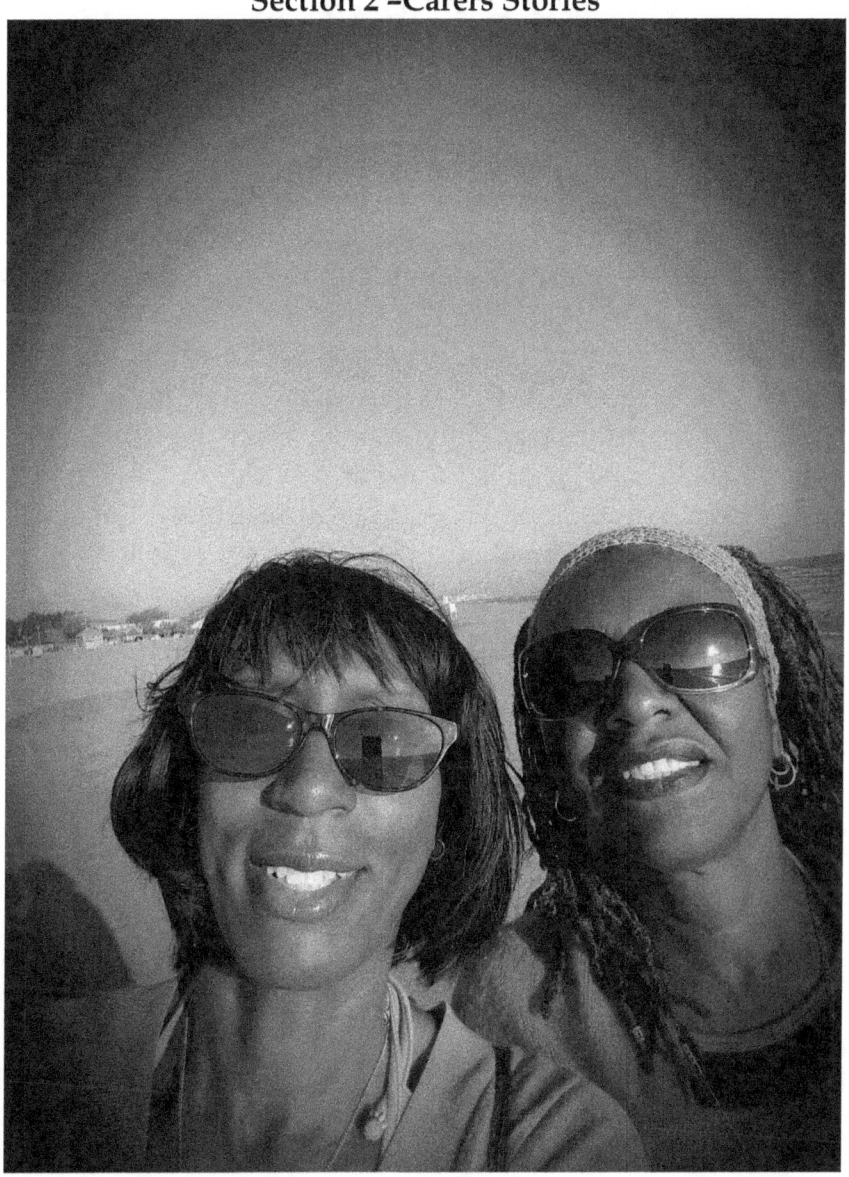

Landa and Rosie

8 ROSIE'S STORY

"She is coming here to steal what I have. She works, I don't work anymore" Essie

There were so many accusations. One of the first was when Essie had said that I took her sheets or duvet covers off her washing line in Kingsmead and I didn't even go to her house.

However, the first major time was when she said I took her plates. I had gone to Ridley market and bought these plates with Elaine, my friend. I invited my mum for dinner the Christmas after. When she came she saw the plates, she was vexed with me at Christmas but she waited until the April. She hadn't been to my house since that Christmas. I was wondering why she hadn't been, so I invited everyone for Easter. Landa had said mum was cussing about some plates she saw here at Christmas and when she came she just started shouting "yes, you took the plate dem!" I don't think we even had dinner that day. She said she saw the plates at Christmas when she was here for dinner. So I showed her my plates. I showed her all the plates I had and she said "Yes that's it, that's my plate!" I thought "Those are the plates I bought up Ridley market. It was me and Elaine that bought them".
 I used to have my friend Wenda's children and so I bought two small ones for the children and four deep ones. It was the smaller ones that she said I stole. I just said ok. She couldn't find the other one. She said I hid it. So I went in my sitting room and went into the unit and took out my set of plates. I said "you can have them, have these, all of them. Just take them"
"No, I don't want them. I want my plates!" she said. So I told her again to come and take the plates, but she said "you stole the other one, you have the other one!" For the sake of -one plate, she refused to take the others. I offered my new set but

she said she didn't want them and that she was going to break them all.

Landa finally got her out of the door but she spun around and came back in. That was the last straw! I had gone upstairs and I said if I come back downstairs and she was there, I was going to throw her out manually. I phoned my Aunt and I phoned my Uncle and I said "listen to how my mum is going on, listen" I asked them "Can you hear her? Can you hear how she is going on?" I said "I am going to throw her down the stairs and push her out the door" but my Aunt said "No, no, no, it's your mum!"

Elaine my friend was sitting there the whole time and she shouted "Rosanna, she is gone!" and so I came down the stairs. But then I heard her coming back up the stairs again, I thought oh no. When I came downstairs she was on the first floor and I thought "I'm going to kick her out the door" My daughter Kandaze was about 9 or 10 years old and I remember her running up and down the corridor crying. I remember Kandaze crying and I was thinking, look at what the child is seeing. From that she couldn't really get close to her grandmother. It affected her relationship with her because her grandmother was making all that noise. She was seeing her mum so upset and all over plates.

I knew mum was sick because she was saying that I stole her plates when I never even went to her house. Something was wrong with her. It wasn't nice being accused and it hurt. I just thought, there is something wrong here. I hadn't been to her house to take her plates. She had accused me before of taking sheets and I thought "How would I get the sheets off the washing line?" I was thinking "Why would I go on your washing line and take your sheets?" She said I took quilt covers off the line. She said she had folded them neatly on the line so they wouldn't crease and I took them off.

After that I realised something was wrong with her. She accused me of lots of different things, but by that time I had stopped talking to her. I decided I would not go back to her house. When someone comes and accuses you, you keep your distance.

The next thing was, when she was in hospital and Landa suggested that we clean and de-clutter her house. I said I was not going back to her house unless there were all four of us there. I turned up and Landa and Lloyd turned up. We cleaned the place, I did the sitting room, Landa did the kitchen, we left the bedroom, and then the following week Landa and Trevor went back and that's when Trevor took the dress.

She was supposed to go on holiday with the club that week but she became sick (with Polymyalgia). I went on holiday with Uncle Dan and hadn't seen her since I came back and she came out of hospital. So when I came back, I was so pleased to see her come past the surgery, because I kept saying I must go and see her. I put everything aside. When she came, I got rid of all the patients, I told her to wait, only two more patients, finished everything quick and tidied up. When everyone was gone Mum came in and said "Where me frock?" I thought, oh, my, god, seriously, she still on about it? Then she repeated again "Where me frock? You take me two frock, me two wedding frock" I was thinking, you got married twice? But she got mad then, because I did not understand her. She sat down, but I told her "I don't want you in here, you need to go". I tried to get her out but she said "Me naw go nowhere, me want me two wedding frocks" So I thought, if you won't go, I will go. So I left her in there for about five minutes. I told my manager she was in there, she was my mum, she was saying that I stole her dress and that it was Dementia. My supervisor went in to try and get her out and she flounced at the woman "Leave me, me naw move, me naw move, no touch me!" My supervisor tried to get mum out gently and said "oh, come on", however mum was not looking at her to read her lips. She just thought the woman came to put her out. I said to my supervisor "please try another way to get her out". Eventually she did.

So from that time I said, I'm not going back to her house. And it's as simple as that. When we are apart we get on good. I meet her on the street. I pick her up. I see her at family occasions. We talk fine, "good afternoon". She comes and she talks to me. We get on fine, but I'm not going back to her house because if I go back there, she going to say that I have stolen something, and everyone knows, I don't steal.

She accused me and said I took rings and watches. We found the rings in the cabinet in the small drinking glasses, the rings were in there. I realised she was sick a long time ago, because I was dealing with that with my dad too. I had come from him that day, when my car broke down, that day she started with the plates. He used to forget where he put things but he didn't accuse anyone. It was a different type of Dementia. He would say, it's ok, it will come.

I had heard of other people with this illness. My friend Yvonne, her mum was the same. Her mum used to say that she stole things. Yvonne didn't live there but when she went there, her mum was always missing something. She didn't accuse the others; she would always say Yvonne had taken it. Yvonne was the oldest and she lived away from her mum. They didn't have a particularly good relationship.

Jean who used to do my hair, her mum had the same thing as well. So I have heard of friends mothers who have accused them. All around the same time, so I could identify with them.

It was just the same trait that they all had, so we identified with one another.

I did feel embarrassed. This one time my friend asked mum about me on the bus. She asked mum whether she had seen me and mum said "No, me no see she, she awa teef!" My friend tried to quieten her but she got even more upset. My friend said "I saw your mum and she was so embarrassing on the bus. She was saying how you stole her things. I was trying to tell her to quieten down but she was not taking any notice, she was just going on, and on about how much you stole" I thought, oh my god. How embarrassing is that? I hope no one else on the bus knew that she is my mum.

And there was Mrs Irish too. Mum went to Mrs Irish and told her that Landa had stolen her nightdress. There were three nightdresses, a yellow, a pink and a blue one. Landa took the yellow nightdress and a hand mixer. Mum went to Mrs Irish the next day and said that Landa stole her nightdress. She even walked with the other two, the pink and the blue one to show Mrs Irish. Mrs Irish phoned me at work and told me to come. She told me that mum was there and accusing Landa. So I went around to Landa's house after work as soon as I saw the nightdress I asked Landa "where did you get that ugly looking nightdress from?" Landa said from her mum. There were a few things Landa took. The nightdress, a clothes rack and a baby mixer because Mum had so many of these handheld mixers. Landa didn't even have a chance to put them away. She came in and dropped them in the passage. When I came, I saw them in the passage way. That nightdress couldn't have fit anyone else
anyway; the only person it could have fit would have been Landa. Landa said that she had asked permission to take those things. Mum came to Landa's house the next afternoon. She had arrived before Landa arrived from work and was waiting for her. Landa gave her back everything and her keys.

Landa then called her brother Lloyd and told him he better go and look after his mother from then on because she was not going back there, she had given back her keys.

That's when the changing of the locks started, around that time. The locks started being changed because mum was saying the work men were coming in.

Landa said that she was not going back to her house. She gave mum back her keys. Landa said she didn't steal and her mum had said she could have those things. Mrs Irish said "Imagine, Essie brought the two nightdresses down here to show me that Landa stole one of them" Mrs Irish said "she's not well. She's just not well"

Essie and baby Landa

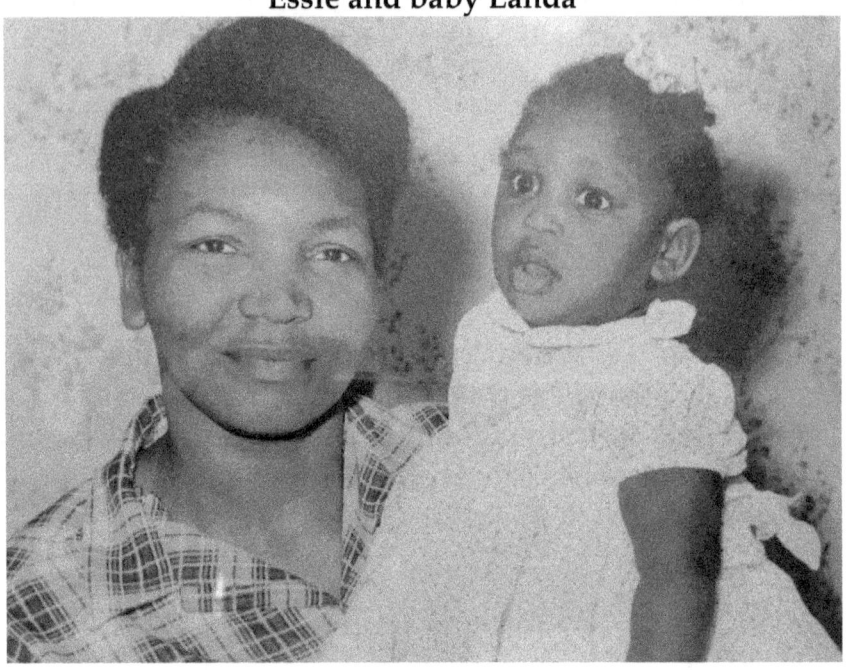

9 LANDA'S STORY

"That big woman, she took my curtains!" Essie

My first experience of Essie's delusions was around 1995, when my Essie was 64. I was the youngest 'child' and the last one at home when I decided to leave home to be more independent. I left Essie living in Kingsmead Estate- a large dark, depressing council estate on the 2nd floor in which she had brought up myself and my brother, Lloyd. As mum was deaf and was not strong in her reading and writing, I understood that she missed not having me around to support her and so I stayed close by, just 15 minutes away and visited every Sunday for dinner and other times when I was passing. It was on one of these visits when Essie showed the first signs of what I now know as a delusional thinking.

In Caribbean culture, the sitting room is a room that is kept pristine and neat. Everything is in place, freshly vacuumed, clean and tidy just in case of a visitor. In Essie's sitting room was floral print wall paper, colourful patterned carpet with rubber backing, black and white pictures of relatives hung on every wall, souvenirs from seaside towns on the fireplace above the electric heater. Taking up most of the room was a burgundy leatherette sofa and two armchairs. On each of these armchairs and sofa were a set of matching pleated burgundy cushions, which were so popular with her friends at this time.

I was having a pleasant visit with Essie. Chatting about this and that when out of the blue Essie told me that one of her pleated burgundy cushions were missing. As far as she was concerned only one person could be the culprit and that was me. At first, I thought it was a joke. Why would I steal a cushion? However, as I witnessed my Essie becoming more and more irate and worked up, I knew it was no joke. She really believed I stole her cushion! She became angry and started ranting about her cushion. Her face changed and she looked like a different person to the person she had been 15 minutes before. The more I denied taking the cushion, the more agitated and angry she became. I was disorientated. This was unexpected and did not make sense, what should I do? Should I help her look for the cushion? Maybe it had got lost. Even if it had got lost, why the big deal, it was just a cushion!

It was then that she did something I was not expecting. Essie always kept her keys in the door lock. She went purposefully to the front door, turned and double locked the door and clutched the keys tightly in her hands. She told me that she wouldn't let me leave. She wanted the return of her cushion. It was then I started to become a bit worried, I needed to get out and now. I looked above the front door where there was a small window for ventilation, and I calculated that was too small to exit from. I moved quickly into the back bedroom which led onto the front balcony. I climbed up onto the large deep window sill, opened the window and shouted to my friend waiting in my car in the courtyard below. However, despite my call, he didn't hear me. As my heart started beating out of my chest, I looked down to see Essie shouting and screaming at me from below. She was becoming more worked up using her arms to express her upset with me and she was now sweating. I knew what I was going to have to do. I wanted to leave but I was also very aware that Essie was in her sixties and I didn't want to hurt her.

I jumped down and attempted to grab the keys out of Essie's hands. However, her fingers just jut tightened further around them as she clutched onto them with an iron grasp. We struggled into the passage and then into the bathroom, me attempting to prise the keys away from her. As we entered the bathroom, I pushed Essie into the bath which was filled with water and the clothes she was washing by hand. The shock of the temperature of water, relaxed her grip on the keys and at last I was able to grab hold of the keys. I ran to the front door, unlocked the bottom lock. I heard mum get out of the bath, as I unlocked the top lock. I opened the front door and ran down to the car.

This was the first time Essie accused me of stealing anything that I remembered. Now, I can reflect that this was probably triggered by loneliness, low mood and the isolation of me leaving home. I told family and friends about this incident. It merely raised a few eyebrows and was then forgotten. No-one thought it was a symptom or the beginning of something serious. Strangely enough, it did not affect our relationship and as far as I remember Essie never mentioned that incident again. It was like it had never happened. Life went back to normal for a bit and then things progressed to the next stage.

In the next few years, accusations became centred around my big sister-Rosanna who I call Rosie. Rosanna or Rosie is Essie's first daughter. They have a difficult relationship which is in part due to separation of 11 years when Essie immigrated to the UK when Rosanna was two years old. The other reason is the fact that they are both rather stubborn!

The second incident involving Essie's delusions was at Easter in the late 90's. Our family were having dinner at Rosie's house. The house was filled with children, noise and activity. In all of that, through turkey and full trimmings mum spotted some plates that looked familiar to hers. Essie started accusing Rosie of stealing her plates and Rosie defended herself.

As I explained above, they had always had a difficult relationship and as a result Rosie was not a frequent visitor at Essie's house and so knowing this, no one took her accusations seriously. We thought Essie was just being difficult. We tried to reason with her. Nothing worked. However, unlikely the theft Essie refused to reconsider. She seriously went into a rage. She started ranting and was unable or unwilling to stop. I remember Rosie and Essie struggling at the top of her stairs, and feeling very scared that someone would get hurt.

Their relationship, which was never that close anyway, just went down-hill from that Easter. Over the next 10 years Essie had a fixed belief that Rosie had a key and was coming into her house and stealing items. These included vests, hats, dresses and others things. Nothing made sense and it was ridiculous to everyone, but still Essie believed it was true. Locks were changed, changed and changed again, but Essie believed that somehow Rosie was getting the new keys and getting in. Essie even went to Rosie's place of work at a doctor's surgery and made accusations and caused distressing scenes. Essie talked to Rosie's friends, acquaintances, explaining in full details and in public her accusations about Rosie's thefts. Rosie felt very angry about the situation. She worried that despite the ridiculous claims, some people may start to believe our mother's accusations. As a result, an already difficult relationship became more fraught and unworkable.

Essie's delusions of theft basically ended their relationship for at least a decade of their lives. Rosie could not visit Essie or speak to her without getting hostile looks or verbal abuse. At every encounter, Essie had something toxic and negative to say about Rosie and it was so painful to listen to. At every visit to Essie's home, family members defended Rosie against Essie's accusations. It led to one argument after another, for years and years. It eventually led to a fragmentation of our family. In a family that is generally loving and supportive, delusions was a poison that affected Essie's relationship with Rosie's two children and grandchildren, who never developed a close loving relationship with their grandmother because of the negativity and anger she expressed towards Rosie. This was the norm for our family for about the last 10 years until the beginning of 2015.

Essie moved from Kingsmead Estate in 1997 to a bungalow nearby. Over the years she developed a close relationship with a neighbour, Mimi. During 2015, we asked Mimi to do some cleaning for Essie because she had been a trusted neighbour for over 15 years, and mum was now getting more frail and needed more support. Mimi did a great job and everything was fine for a few months, until the accusations began. Essie started complaining that Mimi had taken food, cutlery, pots, pans, clothes. The accusation started slowly and then they just became overpowering. Essie just went on and on. She was distressed, angry and tearful. She wanted her locks changed, again. She wanted us to report the "thefts" to the police and harassed Mimi asking for her 'stolen' items back. Essie even searched Mimi's house in the early hours of the morning and upset Mimi and her children. As a family, we found it very difficult. I knew Mimi had not taken the items. I knew Essie was upset. I tried to be supportive to both Essie and Mimi. However, when Essie saw me talking to Mimi, she felt betrayed.

In the last 6 months of 2015 Essie's delusions became very acute. She was complaining of insomnia, she was tearful and the psychiatrist even suggested she expressed feelings suicidal. We were working with her consultant, mental health nurses and GP to ensure we were doing all we could with medication to reduce symptoms. We increased our level of support to her and were seeing Essie most days. I feel for Essie, she really believes the things she says are true and nothing in the world will ever convince her otherwise.

10 MIMI'S STORY

"She works for the council. She works for enough money. Why does she steal from me? I'm not working anywhere"
Essie

I knew Essie a long time before she started accusing me and I knew she already had this issue of accusing other people. She had Dementia and always kept repeating the same things. So when she accused me at first, I did feel disappointed. On top of that because we knew her as Co Co Essie or grandma in this house so we didn't have a choice.

Even the kids asked "Mummy, is it right that Coco Essie has been accusing you of stealing her stuff" I said "Yes" Now she keeps saying things to everybody. When she sees me she always shouts, stops me in the road and is telling neighbours. Yes, I was really down.

She was accusing me in the house, pointing and saying "you, you you!" but because we knew her, we ignored it, because it was Coco Essie. I thought, if she was accusing even Rosanna, her daughter from years ago, then why not me? So I took it as normal. This is now. Rosanna is resting, now it is my time, yes, now it is my time. I became more upset because when the older neighbours came to know, they would be stopping me and telling me, you know that Essie is saying this and that but we understood that she was not herself. She has a mental problem and she has Dementia. She cannot forget the things from years ago, she remembers and has them in her head, but the things we want her to know, she doesn't want to know. She knows the things from years ago.

47

I came to realise from my training, that this is part of Dementia. She kept going on and on. The repetition is caused by changes that happens in the brain. It was really, really good work experience for me. I had training because I am a volunteer in the community. They always offer us training because they know that we go to visit the older people and we must know how they act and how they talk. If someone has Dementia, other problems or a mental issue, we learn how to deal with them and how to make them calm down, things like that. So that is why I was trying, because she was really one of us at home. I knew that with me, she was going to calm down because she knew us properly. I thought it was going to be ok…but anyway, it ended up like this.

It happened all of a sudden, the first time, I was not at home. I didn't know. When I came in the kids said Coco Essie was here. Why? because she saw the bag, the old clothes we were sorting out with her. She saw one very old style green bridesmaid dress, for a wedding. When we were sorting with her, she said it could go to charity, so I don't know if she forgot that these were the clothes we sorted for the charity. I left the bag in my corridor and she saw it. Yes and when I came in that night, the bag had gone, she took the bag. From then on, everything got worse.

After that she kept thinking that her sugar was lost, "oh my spaghetti, oh my this, oh my that, oh my suitcase!". So many different things, she lost. She said I broke her suitcase too, the lock. She used to say that Rosanna broke the lock when she came over but suddenly now that changed and now she said I broke the lock and took the key. So many things were going on and still going on.

So now I am the target. At least Rosanna can rest, it is me now. We don't bother anymore, we know how she is. It really affected the kids, because they couldn't believe that Coco Esther could say these things about me. They heard her say, that I am a thief and a lair, she would shout, she would stop me in the road. I told the children that when they see her, always greet her and say "Hello Coco Esther" to see if she is against them. Sometimes she ignores them and sometimes she responds to them and stops to talk, but for me, no friendship, no nothing.

I remember long ago, we called the police on Essie's behalf. When the police came they said "we can't see anywhere the thief has entered, unless it was a ghost" This was when she was saying things were getting lost, so at that time the police came to search, they looked and could not see anything to report to confirm that a thief had entered the house. The police said it must be because she is old or it must be ghosts because no one else has entered the house. Later on she said she would call the police for me and I said to her "you know what, if you want to call the police, call them. I am a victim, you call them" After that nothing, I didn't hear anything.

Essie could be coming along calmly and then when she sees me she shouts "you have taken my coat!" Last week it seemed like it is coming back a bit. When she sees me outside, she opens up her gate "I will take you to court!" "I will take you to court!"

I wasn't sure if people believed her, because you never know people's hearts and what people are thinking. But I know they knew something was wrong already. A long time ago as they knew me, they came to talk to me. Sometimes when they passed the neighbours could hear Coco Esther shouting with herself inside the house. Sometimes they came to ask me about Coco Esther talking to herself and I said "this is Coco Esther from a long time ago". She could be there by herself and you would think she has a visitor but she is shouting for no reason for the things that are old, old stuff. They eventually came to understand.

11 LLOYD'S STORY

"She takes my sugar, my coffee, my rice, my soap powder. No matter what I put here, she takes it. What does she do with her money?" Essie

The first experience I remember of mum accusing someone was when she was at Malmsmead House (Kingsmead) when she claimed that someone was stealing her clothes off the washing line. She was accusing neighbours and people like that but eventually she got around to accusing Rosanna. It was not far-fetched, people can and do things like that especially in an area like that. When Rosanna was initially accused, I felt really bad for her because at that stage in our family I felt that it was a time as adults when the rift between mum and Rosanna should have improved and it was improving, but then when mum started accusing her, I didn't think it was fair on Rosanna. But one thing for sure, that was the first time I knew something was definitely wrong. I knew something was wrong because I knew Rosanna wouldn't do that. It was a bit stupid. How could you accuse someone, regardless of whether it was happening or not? Would someone go all that way from one area to another to steal something as trivial as a bed sheet? And off a washing line at that! I knew something wasn't right.

Initially, I would tell mum she was being silly and she would move on. Later on, no matter what was said it would always come back to that point. In fact it got worse because the same incidences would often appear each time I spoke to mum a week or a month later, the same incidence would come up again. It got really bad when she moved where she is now.

At one stage, yes I believed her. The reason I believed her was, it was too many coincidences. There were too many things going missing over a period of time. I thought maybe someone was preying on the old woman and they had a key. Maybe they were coming in and maybe instead of ransacking the place, just taking the odd thing so they could come back a month later and take something else. Because she is an old woman and nothing had been ransacked she didn't necessarily know that someone has been in there. That was my thought, which is why I changed the locks as mum asked. I have changed the locks about three times and then I just started changing the keys- about four times. It helps for a little while and then you are back to square one. Mum wanted to lock her internal doors but I've never agreed with that because of safety.

Normal visits were a bit strained because I went there to see my mum and before mum would say how are the kids? or how's this and that? We would talk about everyday things. What did you do this week, what you got planned for next week? We would talk about how things were in Montserrat. It became that the subject always get back to this person or that person taking something. It made it so bad that you just wanted to get out of there. No matter what you did to try and change the subject, sometime it would go back to the same thing. You would just forever spend your time saying to her "No she didn't take it!" "You made a mistake" "You sure you haven't put it somewhere or lost it?" To no avail. It was never resolved. She would just never believe what you were trying to tell her. What would happen is that I would start getting upset and probably raise my voice a little bit and that would calm her down or stop her but it would probably also upset her.

The fact that I was not believing her. I couldn't win. All I was trying to do was to relieve the tension in the family. I always felt in the middle. I would have loved to have been in the position that if she felt something was missing, I would have liked to have been able to help. It got to a point when I felt, if I could have gone into her bedroom and searched and found the stuff then that would have helped both of us. But it never got to that stage. I knew it was a constant battle, so it was pointless me doing that. Anyway, it could have worked the other way because if I didn't find it, then that would be just adding fuel on the fire and she would have said "See, I told you!"

I was hoping that if she found the missing stuff it would make her question herself. "If Lloyd has found that watch that I claimed went missing years ago stolen by someone, then maybe I need to think about all the other things that may have gone missing, maybe I have misplaced them". That's what I was hoping.

You spend most of your visit, battling with her, saying to her "It didn't happen" "No they wouldn't do that!" and she just wouldn't move on. And every visit it would be going back over what you have previously said one or two visits before that.

I went there one day and I was ringing the bell. There was no answer so I opened up the door and went in. I pulled open the living room door and I stood there and mum was talking to 'someone' opposite. Really arguing, putting her case across and then the minute I caught her eye and she saw me, she just cut off, straight away.

I think she has an imaginary friend and it is her way of dealing with her situation and having someone to talk to even though there is no one there. It is her way of getting her frustrations out maybe. She spends an awful lot of time by herself and when you spend time by yourself your mind begins to wander and play tricks on you.

No, I didn't talk to anyone else. I assumed it was an isolated incident with our family. I don't know whether it was embarrassment or whatever. I spoke to my immediate family about it. In a way I kinda thought it was funny and maybe that was my way of dealing with it. Ah she's accusing Rosanna, ha, ha again!

It definitely fragmented the family, without a doubt, especially the big incident that we went through. When we cleared out her house. I thought it was ironic that, of all her children Rosanna and Trevor should get the blame. Landa and I never. I kinda realise what it is. It probably harps back to the past, when Dad and Trevor left and it was just me and my mum for an awfully long time. I think she still has that bond. Not so much now, but the thing is that her mind is still probably back in the past in that sense in that she still thinks that my little Lloyd he would not do that. Whereas Landa is more in the now times and is dependable now. Whereas back then she was dependent on me and I was dependent on her. Like Landa is now, I was her eyes and ears. I read her letters and did things for her then and she looked after me the way a mother does. That's why I never got the blame.

That wasn't a nice time. What made it worse was that we were all trying to help and Rosanna especially Rosanna, she didn't have to, but she went out of her way to help and that's what happened and it wasn't fair again. That was the worse.

I realise now. We know what's wrong and we can't do an awful lot about it. It maybe makes it easier for us to cope with it. It's part of the rigors of everyday life, you can't give it as much time and effort as you would like to. It helps to know her condition but we still can't help as much as we'd like because she really needs constant visits and reassurance. So really I would say the ones that are helping her the most are probably her friends that live close by.

12 LITSA'S STORY

"I'm going to report her to the police. She has done plenty to me but I haven't said anything cause I don't want my pressure to go up" Essie

I got to be friends with Essie through her neighbour Robert who lived next door to her. I met him and I was passing one day and she was at the front door and I started chatting to her and brought her around. We have been friends ever since.

Essie used to talk about Rosanna. She didn't like her at all. She said Rosanna was a thief. She took her clothes, and this and that. Afterwards she started accusing Mimi. Essie said after that Mimi took everything from there, her saucepans and her clothes. Essie thought that Mimi replaced the stuff she took with old stuff in her house. Every other week she brings the whole bag with the rubbish here. I said to her "You bring the same ones, Esther all the time, so why" She said "She come, she took my rice, she took my oil". I go and buy it again for her and she still comes. I said to Essie, your son he changed the locks, nobody can go there. Your daughter and your sons, they have a camera. They can see you in the house and who comes and who goes. If they ever saw Mimi, if they saw her, they would come straight to you. To find out what she is doing there, because they know that you and her don't get along.

Anyway, if I leave Essie in here or in the kitchen and I go in my bedroom to do something or shower. We hear her shouting, really loud. The other day Bonnie was scared. He thought something had happened to her. He went to her and she didn't see him because she was going full speed.

"Esther, Esther, Esther what happened?!" Bonnie asked

"Mimi, Mimi, Mimi she just come and gone, she stole my stuff!" Essie said.

"You are in Litsa's house, there is no Mimi here" Bonnie said

"No! she come, she come. I see her going! Now she is going to my house! You scared her and now she's gone to my house, I have to go and look" Essie said

I said to Esther, "nobody can go to your house. Nobody has a key, only your children, so take that off of your head". So in one minute, she is alright, but if we leave her on her own again, she will start. She will be talking to herself. She is fighting with herself.

She is worrying about me a lot. If anything happens to me, what is going to happen to her. She is with me every day. She said I don't want you to die and she has to kiss me every night. When she comes and when she goes she kisses me. I cuddle her in my arms. They are like babies, when they come to this age. But I really appreciate her, she has been good to me and I have been good to her.

When she gets upset, I sit next to her and I put her in my arms. I rub her back and I say "There's nobody there, you are alright. You are in my house. Nobody goes into your house, forget it"

"She goes, she goes!" Essie says

"Nobody goes there" I say and eventually she calms down and she is alright. She goes home and picks up all the rubbish and she brings them to me again! But we should respect our elders because it is an illness.

When she is upset, she moves her hands, she is really loud and it is scary. It is scary the way she fights. Up to now she is doing it. If I have to go to her house, I listen from the kitchen window and she is fighting with herself. I don't go in though. I just come to the door. She sees Mimi there, always Mimi now. It doesn't make me upset, because if it was my mum, I would take it, so what's the difference my mother or her? It's the same thing. I love her and I try to help her as much as I can.

Anywhere I go, I take her with me. When I go over there to the hall, I'm always taking her with me. If I'm going to the dentist, I take her with me. It's a company for me and for her to get out.

Section 3 –Management of delusions of theft

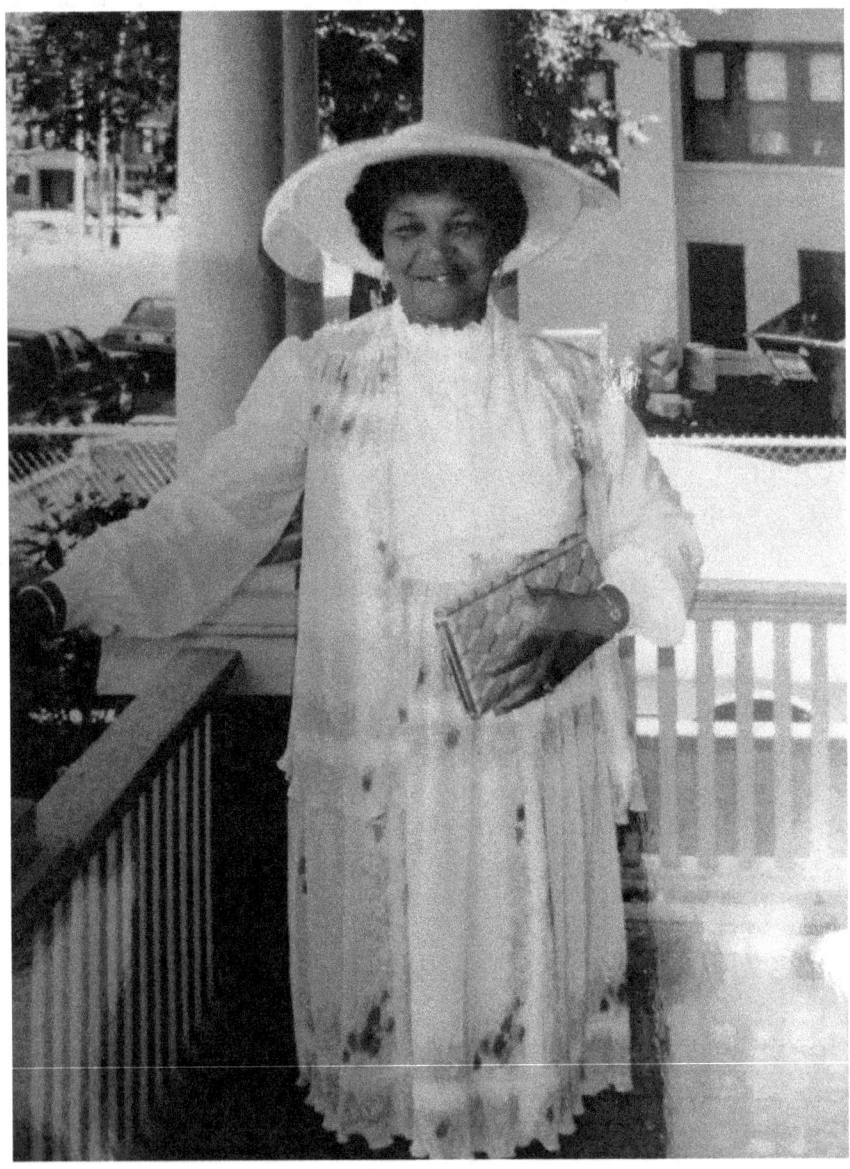

13 WHAT DOES NOT WORK!

"I'm going to tell her to stop this. I'm going to tell the Social Worker" Essie

In this section, I will provide strategies for carers with the difficult task of managing the psychological distress and difficult behaviours associated with delusions of theft. In some cases, the occurrences of delusions of theft may be reduced by addressing unmet social needs or environmental issues like lighting or de-cluttering. These may involve some adjustments, but the benefits in improved sense of well-being for the older person and carer will be worth it and may result in reduced disorientation, improved mood and reduced stress. Any changes should be person- centred and ensure the best interests of the older person are primary. The person with Dementia should, wherever possible, retain some sense of control, choice and autonomy throughout.

In addition, I have included strategies which I have used personally to cope when Essie has been most agitated and upset. I have found that distraction works best at the onset of a rant, as once Essie gets into her stride there is no stopping her! Once highly distraught, I have found that a change of location works well, for example a trip to the

shops or a walk. As exercise is proven to release endorphins, a walk if the older person is mobile may very well have a calming effect.

Lastly, I have included suggestions to increase resilience of carers to enable them to reduce stress levels and continue to provide care. In my professional career working with carers,

I understand that they carry a tremendous amount of emotional, physical and sometimes financial responsibility related to their caring role. This results in stress that can negatively impact their relationships, work, health and quality of life. Therefore, I would advise that on a regular basis carers need to actively focus on their needs in order to reduce the possibility of carer burn out.

Firstly, prior to outlining my suggestions of actions to improve quality of life for older person, I will outline some mistakes that I and others have made in the past that do **not** help people who experience delusions of theft. Here we go:

Don't automatically assume accusations are untrue until they have been proven to be highly unlikely, improbable or false.

Don't try to convince the person with Dementia they are wrong- By definition delusions are fixed and strongly held beliefs that persist **despite** any evidence you can ever provide. Arguments get heated, everyone gets upset and in the end nothing changes. Additionally, research shows that challenging delusional beliefs may make person with Dementia believe more strongly.

Don't shout at your loved one. They are already upset and they believe that someone is invading their personal space, their home and taking their prized personal belongings. In their mind, they are a victim of a crime. Remember they are vulnerable and that they have no control over what they believe. Shouting at someone when they are unwell, is never the right thing to do, despite how upset you get.

Don't tell them they are stupid or silly- Putting the person down will make them feel more vulnerable, worried and stressed. This may make the delusions worse plus make them feel unhappy. When they are unhappy and stressed the delusions are likely to get worse.

Don't agree and go along with false beliefs for an easy life- This may make the delusion worse and possibly work them up into a frenzy. Try however difficult to take a neutral stance. Be supportive but unconvinced.

Don't call them a liar- If you are personally attacked, it may be difficult to contain your emotions, but don't respond negatively. It will be challenging but try to remain calm. If you feel yourself getting angry or becoming impatient, attempt to remove yourself from the room for a few minutes or make an excuse and leave quickly rather than getting into an argument. People feed off each other's emotions, so as you get hot under the collar they will get more heated too and this will not help.

Don't take things personally- Remember that this is not a personal attack, it is an illness. We have seen that delusions are fixed and unshakeable and it is just a waste of energy stressing over it. When you cannot change a situation, focus on changing the way you look at it. Lighten up when you hear about new items you have "stolen". Seek support from family, friends or our online forum at www.theftdelusion.com

14 HOLISTIC STRATEGIES

"I need some shampoo, she stole my shampoo. She went and took it. If she wants one, why doesn't she buy it? If she asked me where I got it from I would tell her" Essie

Every person is a unique individual and what works for one person may not necessarily work for another as personalities, relationships and home situations differ. Therefore, adapt the below suggestions to be person centred care for your loved one. For example, if the person with delusions of theft is not a pet lover, then getting a pet because it is a suggestion may not help. However, if they have in the past derived comfort from a pet and it may help reduce isolation, then that may be a good step. If you are a carer but not the 'accused' person then you will be able to work alongside your loved one to try some or all of the strategies below to reduce the frequency and intensity of delusions. If you are the 'accused person' then this will make implementing some strategies more difficult if your loved one is suspicious of you. If you come up against a lot of resistance then adopt the strategies that you can and focus more on the strategies at the end of this section for carers.

Environmental

De-cluttering- Hoarding is a growing issue in our society today and can have a negative impact on the way an older person utilises their home. It can increase the risk of items being mislaid and as a result increase the likelihood of accusations when missing items cannot be found. You can support your loved one by helping them order and de-clutter their home so that important items can be found easily. De-cluttering may be one way to reduce the stress of people with declining memory who lose items on a regular basis. However, you must ensure that you get your loved one on board with the idea. De-cluttering can cause emotional upset to a person with Dementia so please consider the following:

- Remove just enough clutter to make their home safe, ordered and organised
- Negotiate with your loved one to leave the most important bits of their clutter
- Consider going at a slower pace, to allow your loved one to continue to feel secure
- Encourage the 'letting go' process by allowing the items to go to a good cause like a charity
- Have an enjoyable activity or distraction planned if they become upset

When items are discarded, attempt to remove them immediately from the location to avoid objects being retrieved at a time when your back is turned. If they are anything like Essie, they will not want to give or throw anything away, even if they haven't used it for decades. They may try to remove items from the bin. We have been through this process a few times with out of date food and clothing and it never gets any easier. However, after the process Essie has always appreciated the effect of de-cluttering.

Improved lighting- As explained earlier in this book inadequate lighting may contribute to allegations of theft when a person with Dementia experiences deteriorating eyesight which happens as part of the normal aging process. Changes in eyesight can make items difficult to locate, especially in homes that are cluttered. It is thought that 65 year olds need 3 times more light and 85 year olds need up to

5 times more light, than younger people. Therefore, it is time to get rid of the energy saving bulbs and give them more light!

Change of location- When your loved ones are really upset and cannot be calmed down, a change of scenery works well and my family have used this strategy to great effect. One day when my husband visited Essie, she was very agitated and tearful about the items she said had been 'stolen' by May. She couldn't be distracted or calmed down and she looked like her blood pressure was going through the roof. As I was at work, I contacted my brother Trevor who was able to take Essie out for the afternoon to IKEA. Essie loves trips out in the car and enjoyed a long walk around the bedrooms and kitchens followed by something to eat. For Essie, there is something about the change in surroundings along with the activity and social contact which enables her to forget her delusional thinking and calm right down. Try this strategy and send me some feedback on how it works for you on www.theftdelusion.com

Pet therapy- If the person you are caring for likes pets but doesn't have any, then pet therapy may be something you may want to consider to improve their quality of life. Having a pet or contact with a pet can reduce feelings of isolation and may help the person to feel more secure. There are also additional benefits for example; stroking cats has been shown to lower blood pressure. Consider this option carefully before committing as you need to think about the long-term care of the pet and find an animal that is appropriate to the living circumstances and abilities of the person with Dementia. If purchasing a pet is not an option, consider supporting the person experiencing delusions of theft to visit friends who have pets or perhaps even a pet shop.

Hiding places- In order to ensure they can keep safe their most precious valuables, your loved ones may develop some favourite hiding places. Find them! Expect these to be a challenge to find and don't expect these to be logical or make any sort of sense. Essie loves hiding scissors and sharp objects under her sofa and she also stores quite a lot of sugar under the table in her living room. She hides washing powder in a different location each week, which makes doing her washing challenging each time. Hiding items makes no sense to us, but knowing where a few of her hiding places are means that if we need a screwdriver, we know where to go! Sometimes the hiding places can be very obscure and so it is important that you find these in quiet times so that in periods where your loved ones are agitated and upset, lost items can be located quickly.

Duplicate items- Some carers have suggested buying duplicate items for essentials like glasses or keys and keep them safe for emergencies. When someone with Dementia misplaces something essential that they potentially use thorough the day, it will be difficult to use the strategy of distraction. Therefore, having two copies of keys or glasses may be a life saver.

If this is something that affects you regularly, then this may be reduce the likely hood of an accusation getting out of control. We haven't needed to do this yet as items claimed to be stolen are normally clothing purchased years ago that we can't replace or household items that are not too important.

However, the nature of delusions can change so we are ready to adapt if need be.

Create a safe hiding place- If you are not the 'accused' person, give your loved one, one or two small, medium or large sized boxes and let them know that this is to keep special items safe.. Having a special place may increase their feelings of security and could help you find items that go missing quickly.

Be aware of any patterns of delusions- Keep a diary of good days and bad days and what was scheduled for that day and who your loved one saw. This may help you identify if there are any triggers for their delusions. Is increased agitation more likely on a certain day or after a period of non-activity. Is it linked to a visit from a particular person or absence of a visit.

We noticed that when Essie's has long periods without social contact she is more likely to be upset and talk about things being stolen. As Essie is deaf, she cannot make contact with loved ones by telephone, listen to the radio or enjoy television programmes. Therefore, five days without seeing anyone is a long time for her, especially as she is a very social person. Once we realised this, we now ensure she has contact with a family member nearly every day and her delusions have reduced in intensity.

Information sharing-Ensure carers and professionals working with the person with delusions of theft have a sound understanding of the issues. Provide information and guidance so they know what to do and not to do in the event of an accusation of theft against them or someone else. An understanding of the issues of delusion of theft upfront may reduce the likely hood of a carer or professional 'taking things personally' and refusing to have further contact with the person with Dementia.

Talking about the issues upfront is also an opportunity to avoid high risk situations. Essie has just started a new service where she visits a volunteers home and has lunch twice a week. A small contribution towards lunch needs to be made, however during discussion we realised there may be a high risk area around exchange of money. Therefore, to reduce the chances of Essie accusing the volunteer of taking money, not giving change etc, we agreed that Essie's lunch money would just be paid out of my own account.

Changing locks-As a response to believing that someone is entering their home and stealing their valuables, many people with delusions of theft will want their locks changed. In order to make your loved one feel safe, I would suggest that this would be a good course of action to take, the first few times. The problem occurs when the feelings of relief last only a short while followed by another request to change the locks a few days, weeks or months later. Then another request and another.

Essie has had her locks changed many times since she lived at her bungalow. First, she believed that local authority workers had keys and were entering her home, then she believed that the perpetrator was her eldest daughter Rosanna and now the accused is Mimi her neighbour. After many lock changes, we have now got two locks which we alternate on request. It keeps her happy and keeps the costs down.

15 SOCIAL ADJUSTMENTS

"She has money and two cars and she has to steal from someone else" Essie

Non- verbal expressions of care- I would suggest that older adults suffering from delusions of theft may experience more feelings of insecurity and vulnerability due to their delusions. There are no ways to change these thoughts but we can do what we can to express our concern and our care. It is reported that 80-96% of communication is non-verbal. Therefore, you can express your support through your presence, touch, eye contact and listening. This may assist the person with Dementia to feel less agitated and more understood. Culturally, we all have very different expectations on what constitutes adequate intimate and loving care. Therefore, you will have to consider which expressions of non-verbal communication works best for your loved one. It may be a hand on the shoulder, a hug or a kiss but even being close and listening empathetically as they express their worries may calm them.

"She is with me every day. She said I don't want you to die and she has to kiss me every night. When she comes and when she goes she kisses me. I cuddle her in my arms. They are like babies, when they come to this age. But I really appreciate her, she has been good to me and I have been good to her. When she get upset, I sit next to her and I put her in my arms. I rub her back and I say "There's nobody there, You are alright. You are in my house. Nobody goes into your house, forget it" Litsa

Support to search- Can you or another person provide help to find lost items? There is a Japanese study which suggests that people suffering from Dementia are less affected by delusions of theft if they have relatives living with them to help them look for lost items. You may not live with your loved one, but could you assist them to reduce the anxiety produced when items are misplaced? I went searching one day for a dress Essie said had been stolen by Mimi. Rummaging through Essie's wardrobe instead I found a plastic bag right at the bottom, wrapped up in another plastic bag. Inside the second plastic bag was a box and inside the box was jewellery and three watches, one of which she has previously accused Rosanna of stealing. When faced with the evidence of the watches and reminded of her accusations, there either was no memory or Essie was not willing to admit that she had been wrong. I will never know which.

Children- There is an energy about small children that makes them the centre of attention in a room. Maybe for this reason, they may act as a good source of distraction and focus, for people experiencing Dementia. Intergenerational care is a new concept, where children and older people are brought together for stimulating activities like games, art and music. Research has shown that intergeneration work can be mutually beneficial. It can increase confidence and awareness of mental illness for young people and it can provide stimulation and enrichment for older people. Like most grandparents Essie loves to see her grandchildren. The trick is to come up with a stimulating activity that fits both needs. The thing that works the best for us is that my youngest daughter aged 6 loves people to admire her gymnastics moves and Essie genuinely loves to watch. Sorted!

Empathise and validate- Acknowledge your loved one's feelings without reinforcing them. Let them know you understand that they are upset and are willing to help. You could express this as "I understand that this must be very frightening and upsetting for you", "That must be awful ", " It must be frustrating when things important to you, go missing"

Increased social contact- Some studies in Japan have indicated the presence of cohabitating families may reduce risk factors of delusions. Some people living alone in certain studies showed significantly higher frequency of delusions. It is thought the increased risk may be linked to a lack of close trusting relationships and reduced social communication. The frequencies of contact that will make a positive difference will differ according to individual needs. In our case, we found that Essie's agitation reduced when we started visiting every day.

Meaningful activity- lack of stimulation and boredom can be a trigger for delusions. Some people with Dementia experience more frequent delusions at times of inactivity. Therefore, keeping their mind active and giving structure to their days can have a positive effect for people with delusions. Essie visits a social club a few days per week, and likes to go shopping. It keeps her active and get her out of the house.

Calming down- When your loved one gets upset and heated, it is best that you don't react in a way that will further exacerbate the situation. I understand this can be very difficult, as I have been in situations where my patience has worn thin however it is important to stay calm. Reassure your loved one that you understand that they believe something important has been taken and that you will do what you can to find the items. Let them know you understand that they see things in a particular way but you don't see the situation in the same way they do. If you are the accused, the above strategy probably will not work so please see "time out" strategy below.

Time out- If you are the "accused" person and are being blamed for lost or hidden items, it may be difficult to stay calm and caring when you are under a barrage of abuse and accusations. If you are able to put some distance between you and the person you care for, try to do so. This won't make the delusions go away but it will give you a break. If you live with the person, try and secure regular respite.

In my family, a long break made a big difference in the relationship when Rosie was accused. My mother has had a long standing delusion of theft focussed around Rosie and during that time Essie always talked about the items she believed had been stolen by her eldest daughter, Rosanna. We still had family gatherings but contact was minimised between mother and daughter during that period to reduce friction and conflict.

Distraction- This is a classic strategy used by carers for dealing with delusions. I have found that distraction works well when Essie is at the beginning of a 'rant' however once she is agitated and upset, it is difficult to move her attention from talking about Mimi and what she has taken. I normally change the subject or ask Essie an engaging question. It helps Essie to talk about an event from the past she can remember like a holiday, which has the power to also lift her mood. Distraction is my favourite tools, it usually does the trick.

Anticipate needs- The stage of your loved one's Dementia will determine how able they are to communicate their needs and how necessary it is for you to anticipate their physical, environmental, emotional and social needs and make adjustments. Most care packages ensure that physical and medication needs are met, but there is less focus on the impact of boredom and reduced social contact which may have a negative effect on behaviour. The ability to empathize will allow you to consider your loved ones life from their perspective, and make changes to improve their quality of life. Think about taking them out for a drive, out to lunch or on a visit to a relative.

Broken record-After an accusation, instead of defending yourself try to just challenge the evidence using a broken record technique. For instance "I don't have a key to your home, so I couldn't have taken that" Gently keep repeating the facts to their responses. "Your clothes would be way too big for me, I didn't take them". If you change your responses, that becomes a discussion, which may lead to an argument. However, if you keep saying the same thing, they should run out steam eventually especially if you combine it with distraction and a time out.

16 PHYSICAL ADJUSTMENTS

"This is not my spoon you know, not mine" Essie

Aromatherapy massage-We use touch to soothe ourselves and it is instinctive to rub ourselves when we get hurt. We stroke babies to quieten them and we kiss our children better when they fall down. Many older people feel hurt, scared and lonely but may have less opportunity for soothing touch as they get older. They perhaps do not have a partner, children may have moved away and friends may have died. If your loved one would appreciate it, a regular hand or shoulder massage may be a way of reducing stress and maintaining the physical contact with people they trust and love. Using relaxing and gentle oil like lavender relaxes minds, calms tempers and promotes sleep.

Exercise-Encourage and support your loved one with Dementia to stay as physically active as possible. Keeping active supports them to maintain as much mobility and independence as possible. Maintaining independence reduces feelings of vulnerability which could have a negative impact on paranoid ideas. Additionally, when we are active our bodies produce chemicals called endorphins which makes us feel good, reduce our stress levels, leading to a calmer state of mind. Endorphins can reduce the effects of low mood and improve sleep. Research has shown that as little as 30 minutes of exercise a day can help with distress, depression and anger. So a walk to the local shop and back, a walk in the park or a quick bit of window shopping may be enough to improve mood. The use of music to get older people active is a very valuable strategy to lift the mood and distract from delusions.

Hydration-Many older people are dehydrated and this can affect cognition, concentration and mood. Yes that's right, being dehydrated can make people grumpy. Drinking adequate amount of water is central to good care and should be encouraged to reduce confusion and disorientation. Essie is never without water close by and I believe it has really benefited her.

Sleep-This is a fundamental for healthy living and a lack of sleep or broken sleep affects how we see and relate with the world. If you find that your loved one is irritable and sometimes aggressive, ask them how they are sleeping. Are they having problems falling asleep? Waking up in the night? Having nightmares? Or worried about something? Increasing exercise and cutting out caffeine based drinks are a good start but if there continues to be difficulty ask their doctor to advise on other strategies that help improve sleep quality.

Eyesight and hearing- It was only whilst doing research for this book that I realised that older adults with delusion of theft are more likely to have sensory difficulties. This is particularly relevant to Essie as she lost her hearing at 12 years old and now her eyesight is deteriorating due to cataracts. As I consider, how vulnerable Essie must feel, I can understand how deterioration in hearing and eyesight for others may lead to feelings of increased vulnerability and paranoia. In order to ensure your loved one's independence is promoted for as long as possible ensure that they have regular eye check-ups and hearing tests. If they have a hearing aid, ensure that the batteries are tested regularly and are actually switched on!

Nutrition - The importance of nutrition for our brains has never been more widely accepted than today. What we eat, don't eat and the quality of our food, affects the quality of our thinking and our brain health. There are many factors that positively impact our brain health but there is growing research on the importance of fats for our brains to function effectively and with it compelling evidence on the value of taking pure virgin coconut oil on a daily basis to improve brain function for people with Dementia. Coconut Oil is even being heralded for its ability to improve brain function for those already in late stages of Dementia and Alzheimer's disease.

As well as coconut oil, Omega-3 fatty acids can be found in mackerel, salmon, flaxseeds, chia seeds, walnuts and spinach. These are now proven to be essential to brain health for each and everyone one of us as deficiencies in Omega 3 are linked to poor memory, depression, anxiety and mood swings.

My interest in this area was sparked by research collated by the Brain Bio Centre in London. Research indicates that deficiencies in B vitamins a play a part in the development of cognitive decline and that supplementation in key areas of a person's diet can prevent further cognitive decline. Evidence highlights the importance of having diet high in vitamins and minerals to maintain a healthy brain and cognition throughout our lives.

The strategy of improving nutrition for improved brain health is an avenue that my family are researching and the evidence is very compelling. We have been looking into the benefits of taking a combined supplementation of Coconut Oil, a plant called Moringa Oleifera and one called Mucuna Pruriens to improve Essie's delusions. However, whatever supplements you support your loved to take, it is accepted that a diet high in non-processed plant based foods will benefit your loved one in every area of their health.

We love Moringa because it is an incredibly nutritionally dense plant with Vitamin B and also with Vitamins A-K in much higher quantities than other fruits or vegetables. In addition, it is packed with Omega 3 and too many good things to mention. Mucuna Pruriens is also powerful because of its anti-aging properties and its positive effects on cognition and mood. I advise that at a bare minimum, you should attempt to give 2 tablespoons of organic cold pressed virgin coconut oil to the Dementia sufferer each day. This could be added to a daily juice of green vegetables and fruit as a way of getting a powerful dose of vitamins and minerals in a single serving. Alternatively, coconut oil can be added to stews, soups or used to cook with.

For your convenience, I have developed a Dementia First Aid pack with these three herbal supplements plus a colon cleanser to improve cognition for your loved one. Please follow this link http://bit.ly/2lGM9xS to find out more information.

Learning and mental activity- There is a range of evidence from a new science called Neuro-plasticity suggesting that the brain has the potential to grow new brain cells whatever age and whatever cognitive decline has already occurred. Scientists say that when someone struggles to learn something new and there is consistent effort that eventually new brain cells develop. Therefore, leisure activities which demand something of your loved one but also are fun are the most effective. The fun bit is crucial, because without the fun element, people are unlikely to persistent long enough to enjoy any benefits and it would therefore not be consistent. An activity like learning to play a new game or learning a seated dance routine, something that challenges but is also fun, may over time improve cognitive function. Many studies have suggested that being mentally active has the power to delay cognitive decline and in some cases reverse it In the short-term however, introducing more fun activities into the person with Dementia routine will have the benefit of keeping them engaged and distracted from their delusions.

17 CARER SUPPORT

"She comes when I am not here and takes things" Essie

"We don't bother anymore, we know how she is. It really affected the kids, because they couldn't believe that Coco Esther could say these things about me. They heard her say, that I am a thief and a lair, she would shout, she would stop me in the road" Mimi

In this section, I will focus on you, the carer, as I believe carers' needs must be addressed because of the invaluable role you play in society in providing unpaid support, care and assistance in its many expressions financial, emotional, physical and practical.

I have been a carer for as long as I can remember. I have supported Essie with form filling, communication by telephone, in writing and face to face, advocacy, medication advice, consumer advice, shopping, travel arrangements, travel buddy, taxi, cleaner, cook, legal advice, personal care, personal trainer, nutritional advice, access to community and medical care, mediation with family and neighbours amongst others things. Below are some of the strategies that I have used to relive stress. Have a look at the following suggestions and see what may provide some relief to you in times of stress.

Diary- As simple as it may seem, journaling or writing a diary is a great strategy to relieve stress. The process of writing the day's events will help you to reflect and release any negative emotions. Journaling can help you to clarify your thoughts and feelings and become more self-aware when you are not coping. It can help you to track patterns in your behaviour, care or routine that precedes difficult periods and records progress and breakthroughs that have been made.

Carer education- Studies have found that being informed about your loved one's condition actually assists carers to increase their coping strategies. It increases your understanding and for some reason being educated about this issue can reduce the burden that caring can place on you. It can give you more realistic expectations on what you can do and what is reasonable to expect from you loved one taking their condition into consideration. I can testify to the power of carers' education. Previous to understanding delusion of theft, my focus was on convincing Essie that people were not stealing things from her which resulted in decades of conflict. However, as soon as I was better educated a weight was lifted from my mind and I was able to focus more on improving her quality of life. The great news is that you have already taken a powerful step in your education by reading this book! If you wish to continue building on your knowledge, register at www.theftdelusion.com where I will be developing my website with the latest information relating to delusions of theft in an accessible format.

Carer respite- As carers we can be so hard on ourselves. Women especially can put everyone's needs and priorities above their own, so we never have time for ourselves. If this sounds like you then try to schedule regular breaks from caring. It helps if you can have a couple of days or a week's break from caring but I understand that this may not be practical for a large number of people. So what I am suggesting is a number of mini respite breaks.

Step one: Think of activities which you really enjoy, that relax you. It may be something that takes an hour, like a massage, hot bubble bath, a lunch trip. Or something a bit more indulgent like a play or a concert. Don't compromise on what you want and be selfish about scheduling it in. It is crucial element of the management plan to take regular breaks as it reduces carer burnout and enables you to continue caring. Your mini respite is something just for you and it doesn't matter if you do it alone. One of my favourites is a sauna as it relaxes me so much and evaporates all my stresses away!

Step two: Schedule it in your diary. It may take a week or a month to find a space but schedule it in and don't cancel it out for anything except life and death emergencies! If you cannot find space, you are going to have to delegate or delete some other commitment to make room for yourself. Do not feel guilty about this, you deserve it.

Step three: Once you have found a slot, make it a regular entry in your dairy. If it's a week respite and someone will be caring for your loved one, you may find this level of respite can only happens once or twice per year. However, if you are having mini respites of an hour or so each time, then that should be a weekly or bi-weekly occurrence. This is essential, no arguments, just do it!

Carer support- For me being a carer is one of the most worthwhile activities for humanity as it can make a positive difference in someone else's life. However, it also puts us carers under a tremendous amount of stress and is a major risk factor in those experiencing poor mental health. Therefore, be aware when you are having difficulties coping.

For example, you may find your sleeping pattern is disturbed, you become irritable or your mood is low. These may be things that some carers just endure, however without attention these can turn into major issues that will eventually affect not just you, but all those around you. So my advice is, don't keep it all inside! Talk to people who will listen, empathise and understand. This may be someone close to you, family, friends or a work colleague. However, if you feel there is no-one that you are comfortable talking with, then join a local carers group or an online forum where you can interact with carers in a similar situation to yourself. You can use this interaction with others to express what's on your mind, your challenges, distress or despair. You can register for our free forum where carers supporting someone with delusion of theft, support each other and share their progress and difficulties on www.theftdelusion.com

If you are a stage further along and are feeling at breaking point Get help. Can you speak to your doctor? Can you access counselling? Is there help available from your council? In the UK, you should be entitled to a Carers Assessment which will assess your needs. Find out from local carers support groups what's available in your area and how you can move your schedule around to access support.

If you need specific support tailor-made advice for your specific situation consider contacting www.theftdelusion.com for a consultation where we can explore the difficulties you and your family are experiencing caring for your loved one. Together, we can develop a holistic and individualised plan to support both of you. I will support you to identify the areas you need to focus on first for the greatest benefit in the shortest period of time. For a limited period, I will be offering a free 30 minute consultation to the first 100 people to register on my new website www.theftdelusion.com So act now! Even if you missed the initial freebie it is still worth registering as I will be offering resources and advice to provide continued to support to carers.

Longer term additional support in juggling work, family and caring responsibilities, can be secured by investing in a Carers Coaching programme delivered by either telephone or Skype. Have a look at www.theftdelusion.com and find out more about how coaching can help you lead a more balanced life.

18 TIME FOR ACTION!

"She is coming here to steal what I have. She works, I don't work anymore, I 'm 85" Essie

Now you have a plan to improve the quality of your loved ones life and reduce the impact, intensity and regularity of their delusions of theft. After reading this book you should now have a greater understanding of delusions of theft and some effective strategies to make a positive difference in your life. Consider the most appropriate strategies and then put your personalised plan of action in place over a period of 2-4 weeks. I would recommend trying as many of the strategies as possible and keeping a record of your progress. It will take patience and consistency but if you start today you will notice a difference in about 4-6 weeks.

Ensure that you look after your mental and physical health during and after this transition period and put into action my suggestions for carers outlined in section three. Remember the care and support you provide to your love one is invaluable and so are you.

Essie's progress

Since putting Essie's individual plan into place in November 2015 we have already seen a marked improvement in her delusions. Essie no longer gets so distressed that she becomes tearful. There have been no incidences involving the police in the last few months and concerned calls from the neighbours have ceased. Essie's sleeping has improved which has resulted in a calmer and more settled personality. This plan is not a miracle cure and so Essie still has delusions about Mimi, but she seems more able to cope with these ideas without becoming as angry and frustrated. Essie has maintained her independence in most things but as she needs more support each day, we are ready to be responsive to her changing needs; it is an honour. She has celebrated her 85th birthday in 2016 and is still going strong. may God continue to bless and strengthen her.

Dementia is a terrible disease, devastating for both sufferers and carers. I would not have chosen it, but it has chosen my family. I am saddened by the effects on Essie, however I am grateful for the opportunity it has given me to develop more compassion, patience and empathy. It has gifted me the skills to make a positive difference.

I find it is inherent in today's society to always focus on the negative, so I invite all readers of this book to do something different. I believe that in every challenge there is always an opportunity for growth and so I invite you to change the way you look at your circumstances. Focus on the positive and all that you are grateful for each and every day.

Your feedback

I am hoping that I have succeeded in accomplishing what I set out to do at the beginning of this book. You should have a greater awareness of delusion of theft after reading section one which describes what it is, how it presents itself and how it impacts carers. Following the personal stories in section two, you should understand how delusions of theft impacts all those around the person experiencing it. I have only included a few of Essie's carers' stories here, but around the world for every person experiencing delusion of theft, there are carers and family struggling to care and support them. In section three, I have endeavoured to share a variety of strategies on managing delusions of theft, some are easier to implement than others but the goal throughout is to address the unmet needs of the person with Dementia and improve their quality of life. I've learnt that behaviour is frequently a response to our environment, whether it is direct or indirect. When we make changes in our environments, the response is that our behaviour inevitably changes. I appreciate that for many of you reading this implementing changes will be difficult, however if we want a different outcome tomorrow, we have to do something different today.

As you implement your plan, remember to stay positive

e and be consistent. No significant change in behaviour occurs overnight. So stay focussed and record your progress as you go. Finally, I would be grateful for your feedback on how your actions have made a difference and how I can improve the advice I have provided for carers. You are welcome to contact me via the "contact us" page on www.theftdelusion.comYour responses are very important to me and every e-mail shall be answered.

The advice given in this book is based entirely on my experiences of caring for my mother Essie, therefore all the strategies may not be a fit for your loved one. If you require a tailor-made and person centred plan developed for the person you care for, please contact me for a free consultation on www.theftdelusion.com

Dementia First Aid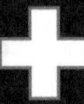

Use these natural remedies improve cognitive function!

- **Organic Virgin Coconut Oil** is a super-fuel for the brain! Coconut oil gives the brain the vital fats it needs to stimulate healing and repair. Research indicates that when taken daily, coconut oil improves cognitive function. Click below for tips on use for cognitive decline.

- **Moringa Oleifera** is a nutritional powerhouse of a plant! Moringa is one of the most nutrient dense plants ever discovered. A well kept secret with everything the body needs to boost general health, vitality and aid healing. Click below for vital information on how this super food can help you.

- **Mucuna Pruriens** can stimulate increases in dopamine which enhances feelings of joy and euphoria. Mucuna improves cognition, our ability to learn, improves mood and feelings of well-being! Click below for details on how this can improve cognitive function.

- **Colon Cleanser**- Our bowels are so frequently ignored but absolutely essential for our health! Click below to understand how neglecting our bowel function can cause disease and how this powerful colon cleanser can re-vitalise your health!

http://bit.ly/2IGM9xS

Need further advice?

- Landa George offers consultancy services in the area of Dementia support specifically the issue of delusions of theft. Services are custom made for your individual circumstances whether personal or corporate.

- With over 20 years' experience of supporting a loved one with Vascular Dementia and delusions of theft, Landa has an in-depth insight into how Dementia can impact carers, families, health and work/life balance. She also has extensive experience of supporting vulnerable people and carers in her role as a Social Worker and registered mental health nurse.

- During initial consultation, Landa will obtain a detailed outline of the challenges you, your family and organisation are facing. Second, she will establish the outcomes you are hoping to achieve. After analysing your unique circumstances, Landa will develop a holistic plan to move you closer to your desired outcomes and improve the quality of life for those with Dementia that you care for.

- Complete an initial enquiry form at http://www.theftdelusion.com/ and Landa will contact you shortly.

ABOUT THE AUTHOR

Landa George is a registered mental health nurse and Qualified Social Worker who has extensive experience of working with older people and those suffering with severe mental illness, specifically psychosis. She also has over 20 years' experience of advice and advocacy work with vulnerable groups.

Landa was a child carer and advocate for her mother who was disabled from childhood. As an adult she has continued to provide care, increasing the level of support provided when her mother was diagnosed with Vascular Dementia in 2009.

Landa lives in London with her husband Colin George and their three children, Cory, Jayden and Maleika.

www.ingramcontent.com/pod-product-compliance
Lightning Source LLC
Chambersburg PA
CBHW070121290526
45789CB00005B/2096